EVERYTHING ABOUT LEUKEMIA

A Complete Guide For Patients, Caregivers, And Healthcare Professionals - Causes, Symptoms, Diagnosis, Treatment, Coping Strategies, And More

DR. CADE JOSUE

Table of Contents

DISCLAIMER

The information provided in this book is for general informational purposes only. It is not intended as medical advice, diagnosis, or treatment.

The content of this book should not be considered a substitute for professional medical advice. Readers should consult with a qualified healthcare provider for diagnosis and treatment of any medical conditions they have.

While every effort has been made to ensure the accuracy and completeness of the information presented, the author makes no representations or warranties of any kind, express or implied, about the completeness, accuracy, reliability, suitability, or availability with respect to the information, contained in this book.

The author disclaims any responsibility for any loss or damage resulting from reliance on the information provided in this book. References to individuals, products, websites, organizations, or other names are for informational purposes only and do not imply endorsement.

By reading this book, readers acknowledge that they are responsible for their own health decisions and should seek appropriate medical advice when necessary.

ABOUT THIS BOOK

"Everything about Leukemia" is an essential reference for those in search of a thorough comprehension and direction concerning leukemia, a multifaceted and potentially fatal ailment. This book begins with a perceptive exposition of leukemia, providing readers with a fundamental comprehension of the disease's essence, attributes, and physiological ramifications. Following this, the text explores the complex classification of leukemia, clarifying the various subtypes and their unique differentiations, a critical aspect in ensuring precise diagnosis and efficient treatment strategizing.

A critical segment of this book delves into the intricate complexities of the origins and risk factors that contribute to the development of leukemia. This section offers invaluable perspectives on the intricate interplay between genetic predispositions, environmental influences, and other contributing factors. Moreover, it provides a comprehensive explanation of the numerous signs and symptoms that are suggestive of leukemia, enabling readers to promptly identify possible indicators and pursue prompt medical attention.

"Everything about Leukemia" provides a comprehensive examination of the complexities involved in the diagnosis of leukemia. It clarifies the diagnostic procedures that are critical for precise evaluation and the development of individualized treatment plans, such as bone marrow biopsies, imaging studies, and blood tests. The following chapters provide an extensive account of the various treatment modalities that are accessible for the management of leukemia. These modalities span from conventional methods like radiation therapy and chemotherapy to more sophisticated interventions such as stem cell transplantation, targeted therapy, and immunotherapy.

Furthermore, the incorporation of a specific section devoted to clinical trials emphasizes this book's dedication to providing readers with knowledge regarding state-of-the-art research and experimental therapies. This enables them to make well-informed choices and gain access to novel therapeutic pathways. Furthermore, this book expands its purview to encompass the critical element of treatment-related side effect management, providing pragmatic advice and support mechanisms to alleviate detrimental consequences and improve overall quality of life.

In addition, "Everything about Leukemia" delves into the psychosocial aspects of managing the disease, placing particular emphasis on the importance of comprehensive support networks and adaptive strategies for patients and their families as they confront the difficulties associated with this illness, in addition to medical interventions. Through the exploration of diverse support networks and the promotion of resilience-building strategies, this book aims to provide readers with the means to confront the emotional, social, and practical consequences that accompany the diagnosis and treatment of leukemia.

In summary, "Everything about Leukemia" establishes itself as an essential resource for healthcare professionals, patients, and caregivers. It provides an extensive collection of information, direction, and assistance that are critical for effectively managing the intricacies of leukemia while maintaining a positive attitude, making well-informed choices, and maintaining optimism regarding potential improvements in prognoses.

CHAPTER ONE

An Overview Of Leukemia

Leukemia is a malignancy that specifically targets the bone marrow, the site of blood cell synthesis, and the blood. This condition is distinguished by the atypical generation of nascent blood cells, which displace mature cells, resulting in a variety of symptoms and complications. The term "leukemia" originates from the Greek words "haima," which means blood, and "leukos," which signifies white, about the profusion of white blood cells that is characteristic of individuals with leukemia.

A healthy individual's blood cells are generated in the bone marrow via hematopoiesis, a procedure that is subject to strict regulation. The procedure entails the transformation of hematopoietic stem cells into an assortment of blood cell subtypes, such as platelets (thrombocytes), white blood cells (erythrocytes), and red blood cells (erythrocytes). An example of the specific function of each blood cell in the body is its role in oxygen transportation (red blood cells), infection resistance (white blood cells), or platelet-mediated blood coagulation.

This regular process is disrupted in leukemia, resulting in the unregulated proliferation of atypical white blood cells. Due to their immature maturation, these leukemia cells are incapable of carrying out their designated functions. Subsequently, an excessive number of dysfunctional white blood cells flood the body, compromising the immune system's capacity to combat infections and giving rise to additional complications.

While leukemia can impact individuals of any age, its prevalence is highest among elderly adults. Although it is more prevalent in infants, this malignancy can also manifest in adults. Treatment alternatives for leukemia differ based on several variables, including the patient's age, general health, and the particular subtype of leukemia. Chemotherapy, radiation therapy, targeted therapy, immunotherapy, and stem cell transplantation are a few examples.

Varieties Of Leukemia

Leukemia is classified into four primary categories according to the rate of disease progression and the specific type of white blood cell that is affected:

1. Acute Lymphoblastic Leukemia (ALL) is a malignant condition characterized by its predominant impact on lymphoid cells, an essential subset of immune-related white blood cells. The condition is distinguished by an accelerated generation of embryonic lymphoblasts within the bone marrow. Although it is uncommon in infants, ALL is a form of leukemia that can also manifest in adults.

2. AML is a subtype of leukemia characterized by its impact on myeloid cells, which are responsible for the production of platelets, white blood cells, and red blood cells. The condition is distinguished by an accelerated generation of undifferentiated myeloid cells within the bone marrow. Although AML can manifest in both infants and adults, its incidence is higher among the elderly.

3. Chronic Lymphocytic Leukemia (CLL) is a malignant condition characterized by the predominant destruction of mature lymphocytes, which are integral components of the immune system. Gradual accumulation of aberrant lymphocytes in the bone marrow, blood, and lymphoid tissues defines this condition. Slow progression is characteristic of CLL, which is more prevalent in elderly individuals.

4. Chronic Myeloid Leukemia (CML) is a malignant condition that exclusively impacts myeloid cells. It is distinguished by the presence of

the Philadelphia chromosome, a particular genetic aberration. A translocation between chromosomes 9 and 22 produces this chromosome, which is responsible for the construction of the fusion gene BCR-ABL. BCR-ABL protein activity is responsible for the unregulated proliferation of undifferentiated myeloid cells. Three phases comprise the progression of CML: chronic, accelerated, and explosion.

Furthermore, uncommon subtypes of leukemia exist, including hairy cell leukemia, a subtype of CLL distinguished by lymphocytes with an aberrant hairy morphology.

Risk Factors And Causes

Although the precise etiology of leukemia remains unknown, numerous factors are hypothesized to play a role in its progression. The aforementioned factors encompass genetic predisposition, specific environmental exposure, and irregularities within the microenvironment of bone marrow. The following are specific risk factors that are linked to leukemia:

1. Genetic factors: Specific genetic abnormalities that can elevate the likelihood of developing leukemia include chromosomal mutations and gene rearrangements. An instance of this is the Philadelphia chromosome, which is linked to chronic myeloid leukemia (CML), and it is formed through a translocation occurring between chromosomes 9 and 22.

2. Environmental factors: There is evidence to suggest that certain types of environmental pollutants, including benzene and ionizing radiation, may elevate the likelihood of developing leukemia. It is known that benzene, an industrial solvent, gasoline, and cigarette smoke, disrupt normal hematopoiesis and increase the risk of leukemia.

3. Prior Cancer Treatment: Certain cancer treatments, including radiation therapy and chemotherapy, have the potential to induce harm to the bone marrow, thereby elevating the likelihood of future leukemia development. This is referred to as therapy-associated leukemia, and it is more prevalent in patients who have received therapy for alternative forms of cancer.

4. Immune System Disorders: Autoimmune diseases and immunodeficiency disorders are examples of immune system disorders that may elevate the likelihood of developing leukemia. These conditions may impair the immune system and white blood cell function, thereby increasing the risk of developing leukemia.

5. A familial predisposition to leukemia or other hematological disorders might augment the likelihood of developing the disease. Certain genetic mutations linked to

leukemia may, in certain instances, be transmitted hereditary from either one or both parents.

6. Age is a significant risk factor for developing leukemia, with the majority of leukemia subtypes being more prevalent in the elderly. ALL is one such form of leukemia that is more prevalent in adolescents.

It is imperative to emphasize that the presence of one or more risk factors does not automatically imply that an individual will inevitably develop leukemia. Some individuals with leukemia do not exhibit any discernible risk factors, and even among those who do, the disease does not necessarily manifest in all.

CHAPTER TWO

Symptoms And Indications

Leukemia symptoms may differ based on individual factors, the stage of the disease, and the specific subtype of leukemia. Common leukemia indications and symptoms include the following:

1. As a result of the impaired ability of the body to convey oxygen and nutrients to tissues caused by the anomalous production of white blood cells, leukemia is frequently accompanied by persistent fatigue and lethargy.

2. The immune system may be compromised as a result of leukemia, rendering affected individuals more vulnerable to infections and fever. Leukemia may be indicated by recurrent fevers, frequent infections, and prolonged illness.

3. Platelet production can be disrupted by leukemia, leading to increased susceptibility to

bleeding and easy bruising. Platelets are essential for the process of blood coagulation. Consequently, those afflicted with leukemia may manifest symptoms such as excessive bleeding from minor injuries, bleeding gums, nosebleeds, and protracted discoloration.

4. Enlarged Lymph Nodes: The accumulation of leukemia cells in lymphoid tissues, including lymph nodes, can result in their enlargement and swelling. Lymph nodes that are enlarged may be palpable or visible in the groin, armpits, or neck.

5. Leukemia has the potential to induce bone discomfort, specifically in the long bones located in the extremities. The intensity of persistent or intermittent bone discomfort can vary.

6. Discomfort in the Abdomen: Certain forms of leukemia may result in enlargement of the spleen or liver, which may induce abdominal pain, discomfort, or fullness.

7. Rapid and unexplained weight loss is a potential complication that may manifest in individuals diagnosed with leukemia, especially in the advanced stages of the disease.

8. Weakness, Pale Skin, and Shortness of Breath: Anemia, which is characterized by a reduction in red blood cell production, may induce manifestations including weakness, pale skin, and shortness of breath.

It is imperative to acknowledge that these symptoms are not unique to leukemia; rather, they may be attributed to alternative medical conditions. If any of these symptoms endure or are accompanied by additional worrisome indications, it is critical to seek immediate medical attention to obtain an accurate evaluation and diagnosis. The timely identification and management of leukemia can significantly enhance the prognosis and standard of living of those afflicted.

Identifying Leukemia

The process of diagnosing leukemia generally entails a sequence of procedures that are designed to ascertain the precise nature of the disease and validate the presence of aberrant blood cells. The following is a comprehensive outline of the diagnostic process:

1. The initial stage in the diagnosis of leukemia entails the comprehensive acquisition of a medical history and the performance of a physical examination. The physician will inquire about symptoms including fever, frequent infections, fatigue, and easy bruising. Additionally, physical manifestations such as lymph node enlargement, liver or spleen enlargement, or atypical hemorrhage will be assessed.

2. The utilization of blood tests is essential in the diagnosis of leukemia. By performing a complete

blood count (CBC), the quantity and variety of blood cells are determined. Leukemia is characterized by thrombocytopenia, anemia, and an abnormal increase in white blood cells (leukocytosis), red blood cells (anemia), and platelets (thrombocytopenia), respectively. The examination of blood smears may also unveil atypical blood cells that are indicative of leukemia.

3. Biopsy and Bone Marrow Aspiration: In cases where blood tests indicate the presence of leukemia, a biopsy, and bone marrow aspiration are customarily conducted to validate the diagnosis and ascertain the specific subtype of leukemia. A catheter is utilized to extract a minute volume of bone marrow fluid from the hip bone during a bone marrow aspiration. To perform a bone marrow biopsy, a minute sample of bone and marrow tissue is extracted for microscopic examination.

These diagnostic procedures aid in the evaluation of blood cell quantity, quality, and stage of development within the bone marrow, while also identifying any irregularities that may suggest the presence of leukemia.

4. Cytogenetic analysis is a method that identifies specific genetic abnormalities in leukemia cells through the examination of their chromosomes. The aforementioned data is crucial to ascertain the prognosis and provide direction for treatment choices. Certain genetic abnormalities, such as deletions, translocations, and mutations, are frequently linked to leukemia.

5. Immunophenotyping: Frequently conducted with flow cytometry, immunophenotyping analyzes the surface proteins (antigens) present in the abnormal blood cells to help identify the specific type of leukemia.

This methodology facilitates the distinction among various subcategories of leukemia, including acute myeloid leukemia (AML) and acute lymphoblastic leukemia (ALL).

6. An examination of cerebrospinal fluid (CSF) may necessitate the performance of a lumbar puncture, also known as a spinal tap, in certain instances where neurological symptoms or suspicions of central nervous system involvement exist. Leukemia cells detected in the spinal fluid with the aid of this test may have metastasized to the brain and spinal cord.

7. Imaging studies, including X-rays, CT scans, MRI scans, and ultrasounds, may be performed to evaluate the degree of organ involvement and identify potential leukemia-related complications, including organ enlargement and enlarged lymph nodes.

After the diagnosis and characterization of leukemia, additional diagnostic procedures may be undertaken to ascertain the disease's stage and formulate a suitable therapeutic regimen.

CHAPTER THREE

Options For Leukemia Treatment

The treatment strategy for leukemia is contingent upon a multitude of factors, encompassing the patient's age, general health, subtype of leukemia, and the existence of particular genetic abnormalities. A combination of therapies is typically employed to eradicate leukemia cells, prevent their recurrence, and alleviate symptoms. The following is an exhaustive summary of the available treatments for leukemia:

1. Chemotherapy serves as the fundamental therapeutic approach for numerous subtypes of leukemia. It entails the administration of potent medications to eradicate leukemia cells or impede their proliferation. Intrathecal chemotherapy involves the administration of chemotherapy directly into the cerebrospinal fluid as opposed to orally or intravenously. To minimize the risk of

drug resistance and target leukemia cells at various stages of the cell cycle, combination chemotherapy regimens are frequently employed. Chemotherapeutic

agents frequently employed in the treatment of leukemia comprise daunorubicin, methotrexate, cytarabine, vincristine, and idarubicin.

2. Targeted Therapy: Drugs that are part of targeted therapy selectively target pathways or molecules that are crucial for the survival and proliferation of leukemia cells, thus minimizing damage to healthy cells. Illustrative instances of targeted therapies for leukemia encompass monoclonal antibodies (e.g., rituximab, alemtuzumab) for specific subtypes of acute lymphoblastic leukemia (ALL) and tyrosine kinase inhibitors (e.g., imatinib, dasatinib, nilotinib) for chronic myeloid leukemia (CML).

3. The objective of immunotherapy is to augment the immune response of the body in opposition to

leukemia cells. A form of immunotherapy known as monoclonal antibody therapy employs laboratory-produced antibodies to selectively bind to particular proteins on leukemia cells, thereby designating them for immune system annihilation. An alternative strategy, referred to as chimeric antigen receptor (CAR) T-cell therapy, entails the genetic modification of a patient's T cells so that they can identify and eliminate leukemia cells. In particular, immunotherapy has demonstrated encouraging outcomes when applied to specific strains of ALL and lymphomas.

4. Stem cell transplantation, alternatively referred to as bone marrow transplantation, might be advised for individuals diagnosed with relapsed or high-risk leukemia. This methodology entails the substitution of impaired or diseased bone marrow with viable stem cells procured either from the patient (autologous transplant) or from a donor (allogeneic transplant). Stem cell transplantation

facilitates the administration of radiation therapy or high-dose chemotherapy to eliminate leukemia cells and reinstate the production of healthy blood cells.

5. Radiation Therapy: High-energy radiation beams are utilized in radiation therapy to destroy or prevent the growth of leukemia cells. It is frequently administered in conjunction with stem cell transplantation or chemotherapy, especially in the treatment of leukemia that affects the central nervous system or specific organs bearing a heavy disease burden. Brachytherapy is an internal form of radiation therapy, whereas external beam radiation is administered externally.

6. Supportive care is an indispensable component alongside active anti-leukemia treatments. Its primary objectives are symptom management, complication prevention, and enhancement of the patient's overall quality of life. Antibiotics or antifungal drugs may be administered to prevent

infections, transfusions of red blood cells and platelets may be utilized to treat thrombocytopenia and anemia, and analgesics and anesthetics may be administered to manage pain, vertigo, and other treatment-related adverse effects.

7. Clinical Trials: Patients diagnosed with leukemia, especially those experiencing refractory or relapsed disease or those interested in novel treatments and therapies currently under investigation, may be eligible to participate in clinical trials. By assessing the efficacy and safety of novel pharmaceuticals, treatment combinations, and therapeutic strategies, clinical trials ultimately improve the quality of life for patients with leukemia.

Treatment decisions are frequently reached through collaborative efforts among a diverse group of healthcare practitioners, comprising specialized nurses, oncologists, hematologists, and radiation oncologists. This approach ensures that the patient's preferences and care objectives are duly considered.

The Use Of Chemotherapy

Chemotherapy is a systemic treatment modality that employs pharmaceutical agents to eradicate malignant cells or impede their proliferative processes. Combining this therapy with others, such as radiation therapy or stem cell transplantation, is commonplace. It is one of the principal treatment modalities for leukemia. A comprehensive synopsis of chemotherapy, as it pertains to the management of leukemia, follows:

1. Chemotherapy drugs function by selectively targeting cells undergoing accelerated division, which includes malignant cells. They induce cell mortality by interfering with numerous phases of the cell cycle, including DNA replication and cell division. Chemotherapy drugs induce a variety of adverse effects in

addition to their impact on malignant and healthy cells, in contrast to targeted therapies that selectively target cancer-promoting molecules or pathways.

2. Chemotherapy Drug Types: The treatment of leukemia involves the utilization of various classes of chemotherapy drugs, each characterized by a distinct mechanism of action and profile of adverse effects. These consist of:

• Alkylating agents, such as cyclophosphamide, busulfan, and melphalan, disrupt the processes of DNA repair and replication.

• Antimetabolites, such as methotrexate, cytarabine, and 6-mercaptopurine, inhibit DNA and RNA synthesis through their ability to mimic critical cellular components.

• Anthracyclines, such as doxorubicin and daunorubicin, which inhibit the synthesis of DNA and RNA and cause DNA damage, are examples.

• Vinca alkaloids, such as vincristine and vinblastine, inhibit cell division and disrupt microtubule formation.

• Topoisomerase Inhibitors: Illustrative instances comprise etoposide and teniposide, which disrupt the functionality of enzymes implicated in the processes of DNA repair and replication.

3. Chemotherapy Drug Administration Chemotherapy drugs may be administered in the following ways:

• Intravenous (IV) Infusion: Chemotherapy medications are administered via vascular injection, which facilitates swift perfusion throughout the organism.

• Oral Administration: Certain chemotherapy medications are formulated in the form of pills or liquids, which are suitable for oral ingestion.

• Intrathecal Administration: Chemotherapeutic agents may be administered via intravenous infusion into the cerebrospinal fluid encompassing the brain and spinal cord in specific instances where the leukemia affects the central nervous system.

4. Chemotherapy regimens for leukemia are frequently customized by the patient's age, general health, subtype of leukemia, and additional pertinent considerations. Combination chemotherapy regimens are frequently employed to reduce the risk of drug resistance and target leukemia cells at various phases of the cell cycle. These regimens consist of the concurrent administration of multiple drugs that operate through distinct mechanisms.

5. Side Effects: Chemotherapy's effect on normal cells, in addition to cancer cells, can result in a variety of adverse effects. Frequent adverse effects of leukemia chemotherapy include:

• Suppression of Bone Marrow: Chemotherapy has the potential to induce transient reductions in platelet count, anemia (red blood cell count), and leukopenia (white blood cell count) due to the inhibition of blood cell production in the bone marrow.

Chemotherapy medications have the potential to induce irritation of the intestinal mucosa, resulting in symptoms such as nausea, vomiting, and appetite loss.

Permanent alopecia, also known as hair loss, may result from the impact of chemotherapy on the rapid division of cells within hair follicles.

Fatigue is a prevalent side effect of chemotherapy that may endure for the duration of treatment and recovery.

• Elevated Infection Risk: The immune system suppression induced by chemotherapy may contribute to an elevated susceptibility to infections, encompassing those caused by bacteria, viruses, and fungi.

6. The implementation of diverse supportive care strategies can effectively mitigate the adverse effects of chemotherapy and enhance the overall well-being of the patient throughout the course of treatment. Possible examples include:

• Pharmacological interventions: Antiemetic drugs, also known as anti-nausea agents, are formulated to mitigate symptoms of nausea and vomiting. For promoting erythropoietin production, growth factors such as granulocyte colony-stimulating factor (G-CSF) may be administered.

- Nutritional Support: A nutrient-dense, well-balanced diet can promote healing and support the immune system during chemotherapy.

- Emotional Support: Beyond chemotherapy treatment, counseling, support groups, and other psychosocial interventions can assist patients in coping with the psychological and emotional challenges they face.

7. Monitoring and Follow-Up: Patients undergoing chemotherapy treatment are subjected to routine monitoring of laboratory parameters such as blood counts, which are essential for evaluating treatment response and identifying potential complications. Prescription modifications to the chemotherapy regimen may be implemented by the patient's disease status, response to treatment, and tolerance. Patients typically undergo follow-up evaluations following chemotherapy to manage any long-term adverse effects or late effects of treatment and to monitor for disease recurrence.

Chemotherapy continues to be an indispensable element in the management of leukemia, providing numerous patients with the opportunity to achieve remission and enhanced survival prospects. On account of individual factors, treatment decisions should be deliberated in consultation with a multidisciplinary team of healthcare professionals, as their efficacy and tolerability may differ.

CHAPTER FOUR

Radiation Treatment

Radiation therapy, also known as radiotherapy, eliminates or inhibits the development and proliferation of cancer cells through the application of high-energy radiation beams. It is a therapeutic approach utilized in the management of leukemia, specifically in instances where the disease has a substantial impact on the central nervous system (CNS) or particular anatomical sites. The following is a comprehensive outline of radiation therapy as it pertains to the management of leukemia:

1. The mechanism of action of radiation therapy involves inducing cell mortality or impeding the ability of cancer cells to divide and proliferate through DNA damage. In contrast to chemotherapy, which impacts the entire body systemically, radiation therapy administers precise

dosages of radiation to distinct leukemia-affected regions of the body, to minimize damage to adjacent healthy tissues.

2. Forms of Radiation Therapy: In the treatment of leukemia, two primary forms of radiation therapy are utilized:

• External Beam Radiation Therapy (EBRT): EBRT entails the administration of radiation from an extraterrestrial apparatus. The patient is positioned on a treatment table throughout the course of treatment, while the radiation beam is precisely targeted towards the leukemia-involved region of the body, including but not limited to the brain and vertebrae. Contemporary methodologies including stereotactic radiosurgery (SRS) and intensity-modulated radiation therapy (IMRT) enable the precise administration of radiation, thereby reducing harm to adjacent healthy tissues.

• Internal Radiation Therapy (Brachytherapy): Brachytherapy entails the localization of radioactive sources within the body near the leukemia site, either temporarily or permanently. By employing this methodology, it is possible to administer substantial quantities of radiation to specific regions while reducing the risk of harm to adjacent healthy tissues. Although comparatively uncommon in leukemia treatment, brachytherapy may be warranted in exceptional circumstances, such as central nervous system leukemia.

3. Indications for Radiation Therapy in Leukemia: Radiation therapy may be employed for a multitude of objectives in the management of leukemia.

For patients diagnosed with acute lymphoblastic leukemia (ALL) or other high-risk subtypes, radiation therapy may be employed to prevent or treat leukemia-related complications in the central nervous system.

• Symptom Mitigation: Radiation therapy has the potential to provide relief from leukemia-related symptoms including pain, inflammation, and compression of adjacent organs or tissues.

Consolidation therapy, which involves the integration of radiation therapy with chemotherapy or stem cell transplantation, can effectively eliminate any remaining leukemia cells and diminish the likelihood of disease recurrence.

• Palliative care: Radiation therapy may be employed in instances of advanced or refractory leukemia to alleviate symptoms, enhance quality of life, and extend survival.

4. Treatment Planning and Delivery: Radiation therapy delivery for leukemia entails the following procedures:

• Simulation: Imaging studies, including CT and MRI scans, are performed on the patient during simulation to precisely delineate the target area for radiation therapy and identify adjacent critical structures that should be spared radiation exposure.

• Treatment Planning: Specialized computer software is employed by radiation oncologists and medical physicists to formulate a treatment plan that maximizes radiation delivery to the intended site while minimizing potential harm to healthy tissues. This may require the application of sophisticated techniques to shape and modulate the radiation dosage, as well as the determination of the optimal radiation dose, number, and angle of radiation beams.

• Treatment Administration: Radiation therapy is commonly carried out in several sessions (fractions) spanning several days or weeks, thereby permitting sufficient time for the restoration of healthy tissues between each treatment. A few minutes is the average duration of each benign radiation therapy session, even though the total duration of treatment may extend over several weeks.

5. Contingent upon the dosage, treatment duration, and site-specific adverse effects, radiation therapy for leukemia may induce both immediate and chronic complications. Frequent adverse effects might comprise:

• Dermatological Reactions: The application of radiation therapy may induce cutaneous erythema, irritation, and dryness in the targeted area. There are instances where the epidermis may develop a sunburn-like reaction or become hypersensitive.

• Fatigue: Fatigue associated with radiation therapy is prevalent and may endure for the duration of treatment and recovery.

Temporary hair loss may ensue if radiation therapy is administered to the region of the scalp or neck.

• Nausea and vomiting may occur as side effects of radiation therapy administered to the abdominal or pelvic region, in addition to gastrointestinal distress.

• Suppression of Bone Marrow: The capacity of the bone marrow to generate erythrocytes may be compromised by radiation therapy, resulting in instances of leukopenia, thrombocytopenia, and anemia.

6. Supportive care measures can be implemented to assist in the management of adverse effects associated with radiation therapy, thereby enhancing the quality of life for the patient throughout the treatment process. Possible examples include:

• Topical Treatments: Lotions, lubricants, or emollient balms may be applied topically during radiation therapy to soothe and hydrate the epidermis.

Pharmacological interventions: Analgesics and pain analgesics, as well as anti-inflammatory and antiemetic pharmaceuticals, may be utilized to ameliorate nausea and vomiting, respectively.

• Nutritional Support: A well-balanced, nutrient-dense diet can promote healing and support the immune system during radiation therapy.

• The implementation of sufficient rest, relaxation techniques, and stress management strategies can effectively mitigate fatigue and enhance general welfare throughout the course of radiation therapy.

7. Monitoring and Follow-Up: Patients undergoing radiation therapy are subject to routine follow-up and symptom and side effect monitoring to

evaluate treatment tolerance and promptly intervene in the event of complications. Patients typically undergo follow-up evaluations following radiation therapy to assess treatment

. Possibility of Combination Therapy: To increase efficacy, immunotherapy may be combined with other treatments such as targeted therapy, chemotherapy, or radiation response, identify late effects or complications, and formulate a long-term survivorship strategy.

In general, radiation therapy is of paramount importance in the management of leukemia, especially when symptom relief or localized disease control is required. Although radiation therapy can efficiently target leukemia cells, its implementation must be meticulously strategized and customized to suit the unique requirements and treatment objectives of each patient, while making certain to minimize adverse effects and maximize results.

Cell Stem Transplantation

The procedure of stem cell transplant, which is also referred to as bone marrow transplant, involves the replacement of diseased or damaged bone marrow with healthy stem cells. Stem cells are nascent cells with the potential to differentiate into every blood cell type. In the treatment of leukemia, stem cell transplantation attempts to substitute healthy cells for malignant ones.

Stem Cell Transplant Types Include:

1. Autologous transplantation involves the collection of the patient's stem cells before the administration of radiation therapy or high-dose chemotherapy. The collected stem cells are reintroduced into the patient's body following treatment to replenish the blood cell supply.

2. Allogeneic transplantation involves the procurement of stem cells from a compatible donor, which may be an unrelated or sibling donor.

Following infusion into the patient's bloodstream, the stem cells from the donor migrate to the bone marrow, where they initiate the production of healthy blood cells.

The Stem Cell Transplantation Process:

1. Preparation: The patient is subjected to rigorous chemotherapy or radiation therapy before the transplant to eradicate the malignant cells and inhibit the immune system, thereby averting donor cell rejection.

2. Stem Cell Infusion: Similar to a blood transfusion, healthy stem cells are then infused into the patient's circulation via a vein.

3. Engraftment: Following infusion, the stem cells initiate the process of blood cell production by migrating to the bone marrow. Typically, this procedure, known as engraftment, requires several weeks.

4. Patients undergoing allogeneic transplants are closely monitored for complications including graft-versus-host disease, organ injury, and infections during recovery. A patient's recuperation may span multiple months, throughout which they may necessitate supportive medical interventions such as blood transfusions and antimicrobial medications.

In certain cases of leukemia, stem cell transplantation may provide a chance at long-term remission or cure, especially for patients with high-risk disease or those who have not responded to alternative treatments. Nevertheless, it entails potential complications and necessitates meticulous surveillance and control by a specialized medical staff.

CHAPTER FIVE

Concentrated Therapy

A form of cancer treatment known as targeted therapy selectively targets malignant cells while minimizing harm to healthy cells. In contrast to the indiscriminate targeting of rapidly dividing cells by conventional chemotherapy, targeted therapy inhibits the activity of particular molecules or pathways that are integral to the survival and proliferation of cancer.

The Rationale For Operation:

Drugs used in targeted therapy can exert their effects in a multitude of methods, which encompass:

1. Certain targeted therapy medications inhibit signaling pathways that are involved in the promotion of cancer cell survival and growth. Tyrosine kinase inhibitors (TKIs), which

inhibit the activity of cell signaling enzymes including BCR-ABL in chronic myeloid leukemia, are one example.

2. Certain targeted therapy medicines are engineered to selectively target particular genetic mutations that are responsible for promoting the development of cancer. Imatinib, for example, selectively targets the BCR-ABL fusion protein that is found in CML cells.

3. Inducing Apoptosis: Certain targeted therapy medications induce programmed cell death, or apoptosis, in cancer cells through the targeting of proteins that are implicated in pathways governing cell survival.

Advantages Of Targeted Treatment

1. With the ability to selectively target malignant cells, targeted therapy mitigates harm to non-cancerous tissues and diminishes adverse effects in comparison to conventional chemotherapy.

2. Enhanced Results: Targeted therapy has the potential to yield improved treatment outcomes, such as extended survival and enhanced quality of life, in certain instances.

3. Combination Therapy: To increase the efficacy of targeted therapy, it may be combined with other therapies such as immunotherapy or chemotherapy.

The Use Of Immunotherapy

Immunotherapy is a form of cancer treatment that targets and eliminates cancer cells by utilizing the immune system. Among the vital functions of the immune system is the detection and eradication of abnormal cells, such as cancer cells. Nevertheless, cancer cells possess the ability to elude immune detection through a multitude of mechanisms. By impeding these mechanisms, immunotherapy attempts to enhance the immune response against malignancy.

Varieties Of Immunotherapy Include:

1. Checkpoint inhibitors are pharmaceutical substances that obstruct inhibitory signals on immune cells, thereby enhancing their ability to identify and eliminate cancer cells. Drugs that specifically target programmed cell death protein 1 (PD-1) or cytotoxic T-lymphocyte-associated protein 4 (CTLA-4) are two such examples.

2. CAR-T Cell Therapy: Chimeric antigen receptor (CAR) T-cell therapy entails the genetic modification of T cells belonging to a patient to encode receptors that distinguish particular proteins present in malignant cells. Once reinvested into the patient's body, these T cells that have been engineered are capable of destroying cancer cells.

3. Monoclonal Antibodies: Produced in the laboratory, monoclonal antibodies can identify

specific proteins on the surface of cancer cells as targets for immune system destruction.

Positive Aspects Of Immunotherapy:

1. In some patients, immunotherapy can elicit durable responses, which may result in an extended period of remission or even complete recovery.

2. Reduced Toxicity: In contrast to conventional chemotherapy, immunotherapy generally elicits less severe adverse effects due to its selective targeting of cancer cells and circumvention of normal tissues.

Trials In Clinical Settings

Clinical trials encompass research investigations that assess the safety and effectiveness of novel medical interventions, such as pharmaceuticals, surgical procedures, and therapeutic processes. Clinical trials are of paramount importance in the progression of medical knowledge and the enhancement of patient care through the evaluation of novel therapeutic interventions and approaches.

The Following Are The Stages Of Clinical Trials:

1. Phase I: In a limited group of patients, phase I trials evaluate the safety and dosage of a new treatment. Determining the maximal tolerated dose and identifying potential adverse effects are the principal objectives.

2. Phase II trials evaluate the treatment's efficacy in a more extensive cohort of patients who are afflicted with the specific condition of interest. These trials serve to furnish initial indications of efficacy and conduct additional assessments of safety.

3. Phase III: In a large cohort of patients, phase III trials compare the new treatment to standard-of-care treatments. In terms of efficacy and safety, the

objective is to ascertain whether the novel treatment is superior, equivalent, or inferior to established therapies.

4. Phase IV trials, which are alternatively referred to as post-marketing surveillance studies, commence after the approval and public availability of a treatment. These clinical trials employ real-world conditions to observe and assess the treatment's long-term safety and efficacy.

Positive Aspects Of Clinical Trials Include:

1. Clinical trials provide patients with access to innovative remedies that might not be commercially available beyond the confines of a research environment.

2. Active Participation in Clinical Trials: Patients make a significant contribution to the progression of medical knowledge and the

formulation of novel therapeutic approaches that will benefit future generations.

3. A comprehensive care approach is maintained throughout the clinical trial using close monitoring and support provided by a multidisciplinary team of healthcare professionals.

4. Possibility of Individual Advantage: Although not assured, engaging in a clinical trial may afford personal advantages, including potential access to investigational therapies that can enhance outcomes.

In conclusion, clinical trials, stem cell transplants, targeted therapy, and immunotherapy are all vital components of leukemia treatment that provide patients with optimism regarding their prognoses and quality of life. By replacing diseased cells with healthy ones, targeting specific molecular pathways implicated in cancer growth, utilizing the body's immune system to combat cancer, or subjecting new treatments to rigorous scientific evaluation, each of these approaches represents a distinct strategy for combating leukemia. To progress leukemia treatment and ultimately enhance patient outcomes, patients, healthcare providers, and researchers must work in concert.

Managing Adverse Reactions

Leukemia is a multifaceted and arduous disease distinguished by the aberrant proliferation of white blood cells within the bone marrow, thereby interfering with the regular synthesis of erythrocytes. This malignancy impacts the bone marrow and blood, resulting in manifestations including lethargy, fatigue, recurrent infections, and susceptibility to injury or hemorrhage. Treatment of leukemia necessitates a variety of strategies, including psychological support, lifestyle modifications, and medical interventions. Presented below is an exhaustive examination of each of the aforementioned concepts:

1. Medical interventions: Adverse effects frequently encountered by patients undergoing treatment for leukemia include but are not limited to fatigue, vertigo, hair loss, and heightened vulnerability to infections. Pharmaceuticals may be prescribed by medical professionals to alleviate these symptoms. Antiemetics and growth factors are two examples of substances that can be utilized to induce the production of healthy blood cells and vertigo, respectively.

2. Nutritional Support: In patients with leukemia, proper nutrition is vital, as the disease and its treatments can inhibit nutrient absorption and appetite. A balanced diet consisting of an abundance of fruits, vegetables, lean proteins, and whole cereals may be suggested by dietitians as a means to promote overall health and facilitate the recovery process.

3. Physical activity is an effective means for leukemia patients to mitigate fatigue and enhance

their general state of health. To ensure safety, it is crucial to consult with healthcare professionals before beginning an exercise regimen, particularly during periods of intensive treatment.

4. Psychological Support: The mental well-being of patients may be significantly impacted as they navigate the challenges of leukemia and its associated adverse effects. Support groups, psychologists, or counselors may offer patients emotional assistance, coping mechanisms, and resources to aid them in overcoming obstacles.

5. Complementary Therapies: Complementary therapies, including but not limited to massage therapy, acupuncture, and relaxation techniques like yoga and meditation, may provide some patients with relief from adverse effects. These methods may aid in tension reduction and the enhancement of one's sense of well-being.

CHAPTER SIX

Managing Leukemia

1. The dissemination of knowledge and education regarding leukemia and its available treatment modalities can enable patients to take an engaged role in their healthcare. Healthcare providers must devote sufficient time to elucidate the disease, treatment protocols, and potential adverse effects to patients and their families using language that is comprehensible to them.

2. Emotional Support: The process of accepting a leukemia diagnosis can induce a spectrum of distressing feelings in patients, including fear, anxiety, sorrow, and resentment. It is of the utmost importance to establish a nurturing atmosphere that encourages patients to openly communicate their emotions and seek assistance when necessary.

3. Despite the formidable obstacles presented by leukemia, numerous patients make an effort to preserve a semblance of regularity in their daily existence. This may entail, to the greatest extent possible, maintaining employment or enrollment in school or work, engaging in social activities, and pursuing enjoyable and fulfilling pastimes and interests.

4. Establishing Practical Objectives: Coping with leukemia frequently necessitates modifying one's aspirations and objectives. Patients may experience a greater sense of accomplishment and purpose by establishing attainable objectives that correspond with their present capabilities and desires.

5. Seeking Professional Assistance: Patients who are grappling with the emotional repercussions of leukemia may benefit from professional counseling or therapy, in addition to the support they receive from family and friends. Therapists

possess the ability to furnish individuals with instruments and approaches to effectively cope with tension, anxiety, and various other psychological obstacles.

Support Mechanisms

1. Family and Friends: Leukemia patients can benefit significantly from a robust support network comprising family members, friends, and loved ones, which can offer indispensable logistical, emotional, and practical assistance. The presence of close family and friends during medical appointments, lending an ear, or providing assistance can have a substantial impact on the patient's experience.

2. Participating in a support group catering to leukemia patients and their families can foster a feeling of unity, companionship, and comprehension. Engaging in conversations with individuals who are undergoing comparable

circumstances can provide solace, support, and insightful information regarding coping mechanisms and available resources.

3. Healthcare providers, comprising oncologists, nurses, social workers, and other medical experts, fulfill an essential function in extending support to individuals afflicted with leukemia during the course of their treatment and recuperation. Establishing a rapport of trust with healthcare providers can promote candid dialogue and individualized treatment.

4. Online Resources: Leukemia patients and their families have access to an abundance of information and resources on the internet. Social media groups, online forums, and educational websites offer individuals the chance to engage in virtual conversations, obtain current information, and discover encouragement and support without leaving the sanctuary of their homes.

Preventive Measures

1. Preventing Identified Risk Factors: Although the precise etiology of leukemia remains uncertain, specific risk factors have been identified, including ionizing radiation exposure, particular chemicals (e.g., benzene), genetic susceptibility, and specific chemical exposure. When feasible, minimizing exposure to these risk factors could potentially decrease the probability of developing leukemia.

2. Adhering to a Healthy Lifestyle: Embracing healthy lifestyle practices, including but not limited to consuming a well-balanced diet, participating in consistent physical activity, maintaining a healthy weight, abstaining from smoking and excessive alcohol intake, and practicing sun safety, can potentially contribute to a reduced risk of leukemia and enhance overall health.

3. Occupational Safety: In sectors characterized by frequent encounters with potentially hazardous substances, adherence to safety protocols, utilization of protective gear, and mitigation of hazardous chemical exposure can contribute to an increased likelihood of averting the development of occupational cancers, including leukemia.

4. When a family history of leukemia or other malignancies is present, it may be advantageous to seek genetic counseling. Genetic counselors are capable of evaluating the risk factors of an individual, imparting knowledge regarding available genetic testing alternatives, and advising on personalized preventive measures and screening protocols.

5. Consistent Health Examinations: Consistent screenings and medical examinations can aid in the detection of abnormalities or early indicators of leukemia or other ailments.

Prompt intervention and treatment are possible due to early detection, which may lead to improved prognoses and outcomes.

In summary, the management of leukemia necessitates a holistic strategy that encompasses the physiological, psychological, and logistical dimensions of treatment. Through adeptly handling adverse effects, successfully navigating the emotional obstacles associated with the illness, utilizing suitable support networks, and instituting preventative measures, those afflicted with leukemia can maximize their standard of living and augment their holistic state of being.

Support networks, patients, and healthcare providers must collaborate to navigate the complexities of leukemia and advance positive outcomes.

Summary

In summary, comprehensive knowledge regarding leukemia is critical for healthcare professionals and patients alike. This multifaceted ailment comprises a variety of conditions distinguished by the atypical proliferation of white blood cells; it impacts individuals across the globe and spans all age groups. Considerable advancements in the field of medical science and thorough research have contributed to substantial progress in the diagnosis and treatment of leukemia.

Remainingly, early detection is critical for enhancing prognoses and treatment outcomes. The utilization of imaging modalities and diagnostic technique advancements, including genetic testing, empowers healthcare practitioners to customize treatment approaches by the particular subtype and genetic profile of leukemia.

The landscape of leukemia treatment has undergone substantial development, although conventional chemotherapy continues to be the cornerstone. Targeted therapies, immunotherapy, and stem cell transplantation have been added to this repertoire. Innovative targeted therapies, which are engineered to selectively target malignant cells while preserving healthy tissues, have significantly transformed the approach to treating leukemia by providing enhanced effectiveness and diminished adverse effects.

Furthermore, current research initiatives persist in their pursuit to elucidate the molecular processes that govern the onset of leukemia, thereby creating opportunities for the advancement of novel therapeutic interventions and personalized medicine strategies. Progress toward more efficacious treatments and, ultimately, improved outcomes for individuals afflicted with leukemia necessitates the indispensable collaboration of pharmaceutical companies, researchers, and clinicians. Fundamentally, despite the formidable obstacles that leukemia poses, the combined endeavors of the medical community provide optimism regarding enhanced survival rates and overall quality of life for individuals afflicted with this ailment.

THE END